I0113254

Our Health
&
The Bible

How To Create A Healthy Lifestyle
With The Word Of God

Alberto Rodriguez

Copyright © (2025) Alberto Rodriguez

All rights reserved.
No portion of this book may be reproduced or transmitted
by any means-electronic, mechanical, photocopy,
recording, or otherwise without the prior written permission
of the copyright owner.

Alberto Rodriguez
Email: Healthyandsaved@gmail.com

Hardcover ISBN: 979-8-218-64863-3

Editor: Abigail Gonzalez

Book Cover Designed by: Simara Rodriguez

Table of Contents

Dedication

Life sometimes feels like a relentless treadmill, constantly running but getting nowhere. We wake up, rush through our morning routines, and dive headfirst into the chaos of our responsibilities. But let me remind you: you have the right to pause. You can reclaim your time, starting with these small moments of stillness.

This book is not just a collection of words; it's a guide meant to help you navigate through the chaos of life. It's about finding balance, embracing your rhythm, and giving yourself permission to slow down.

Together, we'll explore practical strategies to enhance your mornings, energize your days, and rejuvenate your spirit. This book was written with **YOU** in mind and written with POWER. I'm here to encourage you to get up again.

I devote this book to those trying to balance fast food and cooking dinner while needing time to go grocery shopping. This is for you. And let me not forget to mention the many sleepless nights because there's too much to do in such a short 24-hour span.

I dedicate this book to you, the one who can't find time or energy to complete a 30-minute workout. But every day, you try. Hold on to your dedication because what I have for you is special near the end.

As we journey through these pages, I encourage you to embrace the idea of self-care. It's not a luxury; it's a necessity.

Consider what brings you joy, fuels your passion, and makes you feel alive. Prioritize integrating these elements into your daily routine. Whether it's taking a moment to enjoy your favorite song, sipping your coffee mindfully, or stepping outside to feel the warmth of the sun on your face, these small acts can make a world of difference.

Take a moment to reflect on the simple act of breathing. Inhale deeply, fill your lungs with air, and exhale slowly, releasing the tension that has built up in your body. Do this a few times and let the day's stress melt away. Each breath is a reminder that you are alive, capable of change, and have the power to shape your reality.

So, let's embark on this journey together. Let's discover how to rise above fatigue, break free from the cycle of exhaustion, and step into a life filled with vitality and purpose. You are not alone in this struggle; we will find the light that shines within. Remember, each day is a new beginning—a chance to rewrite your story and embrace the possibilities that await.

Don't feel ashamed if you're anything like how I used to be; the list may look like this (list below), but hang tight. We are getting ready to change all that.

*Large loads of laundry that need to be washed or put away

*The workload you keep putting off by giving your boss a new excuse or reason as to why it's not turned in yet

*Having to cook dinner because no one wants leftovers three days in a row

*Caught slacking on spending time with your wife or husband because they should "*understand*"

*The list goes on......what would you add?

How does that work for you who live your life by routine? Do you add anything beneficial to your life by keeping *that* routine? Or do you find yourself watching the lives of others and seeing them enjoy the fruits of their labor?

Many find their chores a daily and even a weekly struggle, and although you may see what needs to be done in front of you, it's NOT impossible to complete when you PULL your strength from the right source. We'll jump into that a little later.

As you progress through the pages, you'll find a series of exercises that challenge you to articulate your dreams and desires. You'll learn the importance of self-compassion and how it can be a game-changer in your journey. It's easy to be your worst critic, but what if you become your greatest supporter instead? This book will help you cultivate a kind and nurturing inner voice that encourages you to take risks and view failures as opportunities for growth.

Remember, this journey isn't about perfection; it's about progress and learning to embrace the messy, imperfect, and beautiful parts of yourself. I invite you to take your time as you engage with this material. Allow yourself to absorb the lessons fully, reflect on the insights, and integrate them into your life at your own pace.

You will be provided with tools to uncover the patterns that may be holding you back and challenge the limiting beliefs ingrained in your mind for far too long.

Through reflective exercises, thought-provoking prompts, and insightful anecdotes, you'll be encouraged to dig deeper into your psyche, exploring the narratives that shape your self-perception and influence your actions.

Each chapter is designed to guide you on a journey of self-discovery. You'll learn to identify the moments when you've been too hard on yourself, allowed doubt to creep in, and let external pressures dictate your worth. It's time to reframe those thoughts and statements that no longer serve you, replacing them with affirmations that empower you to reach your true potential.

By the end of this book, I hope you have developed a deeper understanding of who you are, what you value, and how to create a life that resonates with your true self. You possess the power to rewrite your story, and this book is just the beginning of that transformative journey.

Let's dive in together and uncover the remarkable person that has always been within you, waiting to be unleashed.

After all, our bodies are the temple where the Holy Spirit dwells. Stand firm if you don't have a solid foundation to start the journey. Soon, you will have a strong foundation for your next step and a better understanding of what happens when we stand firm on Him (GOD).

To My Wife,

Kamora, I dedicate this book to you. You are my anchor and safe haven. Your unwavering support has been my guiding light, illuminating the darkest paths and reminding me that love conquers all. Together, we've weathered storms and celebrated triumphs, and through it all, you have shown me the true meaning of partnership.

In every laugh we've shared, every challenge we've faced, and every quiet moment spent together, I have realized how deeply intertwined our lives have become. You inspire me to be a better man and to strive for greatness, not just for myself but for us. Your strength and resilience motivate me to push beyond my limits, to dream bigger, and to embrace each day with gratitude.

Your laughter fills our home with joy, and your kindness touches everyone you meet. I am endlessly grateful for the memories we've created and excited for all the adventures that lie ahead. Together, let's continue to grow, learn, and thrive, hand in hand, heart to heart.

No words can ever express how much I love you! In sickness and health, in good times and bad, we are each other's ride or die. I love you, now and always.

To My Children,

Simara and Gabriel, you are the light of my life and the driving force behind my aspirations. Watching you grow and navigate the world fills my heart with immeasurable pride and joy. Each moment spent with you is a treasure, and I cherish the unique personalities and talents that make you both so special. Your laughter is music to my ears, and your dreams inspire me to reach higher and strive harder.

As your father, I want to instill in you the importance of holistic well-being. Life is a journey that encompasses not just our physical health but also our mental and spiritual well-being. Remember, taking care of your physical health is vital and equally important as nurturing your mind.

Spiritually, I urge you to find your purpose and connect with something more significant than yourselves. Through faith or personal reflection, allow your spirit to flourish. Embrace moments of stillness and gratitude, for they will ground you during life's challenges.

Let's set goals as a family. Let's share our dreams, support one another, and celebrate each milestone, no matter how small. Whether trying new activities, cooking healthy meals together, or simply taking time to talk and connect.

Let's elevate our overall health and happiness as a unit. I am committed to being the best father I can be, which means leading by example. I want to show you that prioritizing our health is not just a trend but a lifelong commitment. Let's create a legacy of strength, resilience, and love together.

Simara and Gabriel, I believe in you wholeheartedly. You have the power to achieve greatness. And while I am here with you, I promise always to support, cheer, and guide you as you navigate this beautiful journey called life.

May our family continue to be blessed, and may we always seek to elevate one another in mind, body, and spirit. I love you both more than words can express!

Introduction

Everyone has one thing they have a hard time with, whether it's going to bed at a decent hour, sleeping throughout the night, getting up early, finding the motivation to work out in the morning, afternoon, or evening, or something as simple as finding the words to pray. Whatever it may be, this book you're holding will help you get to where you want to go.

The number one question I get is, *HOW*? How do we make these things go from the reality of our minds to the reality *in* this world? How do we stop saying what we want and start living out what we want?

The journey from desire to reality begins with belief—faith in yourself, faith in your abilities, and faith in the process. It's about transforming your thoughts into actionable steps that align with your deepest aspirations. Here's how to make our dreams tangible, one step at a time.

1. Define Your Vision: Take a moment to understand what you want truly. Please write it down. Habakkuk 2:2 says, "Write the vision; make it plain on tablets (paper) so he may run who reads it." English Standard Version Bible.
Visualize it and let it become clear in your mind. What does success look like for you? What emotions do you want to feel? By gaining clarity on your vision, you set the stage for transformation.

2. Set Intentional Goals: Break down your vision into specific, achievable goals. Instead of saying, "I want to be healthy," specify what that means for you. It could be exercising three times a week, cooking at home more often,

or meditating daily. Setting measurable goals helps create a roadmap for your journey.

3. Take Small, Consistent Actions: Consistent action is key to progress. Start with small, manageable steps and gradually build up.

4. Cultivate a Growth Mindset: Embrace the idea that challenges and setbacks are part of the journey. Begin to view obstacles as learning opportunities instead of allowing fear or self-doubt to hold you back. This will empower you to persist and adapt as you work toward your goals.

5. Surround Yourself with Support: Share your goals with those who uplift and inspire you. Allow them to hold you accountable.

6. Practice Faith in Action: Faith is not just a belief; it's a verb. It involves taking steps forward even when the path isn't clear. Trust that your efforts are guiding you in the right direction. When facing uncertainty, keep in mind that growth often happens outside your comfort zone.

7. Celebrate Progress: Acknowledge and celebrate each milestone. Every step you take showcases your dedication and effort. Celebrating progress enhances your motivation and strengthens the belief that you are getting closer to your desired reality.

8. Reflect and Adjust: Regularly reflect on your journey. Are your actions still aligned with your goals? Are there areas where you need to pivot or adjust your approach?

Reflection allows you to stay connected to your purpose and make necessary adjustments along the way. By integrating these steps into your daily life, you will find that the gap between what you want and what you experience begins to close.

Remember, the journey is as important as the destination, and every step taken in faith brings you closer to manifesting your dreams.

Reading this book, you will understand how to take control of your health and release yourself from the addiction of pleasing people. Oh, hang tight. I'm taking you on a ride. While you go through this release process, you will also learn the importance of putting God first and not settling for a mediocre lifestyle.

What a good time to understand your health and The Bible, creating the hope and faith needed to prove to YOURSELF that you can live the healthy lifestyle that others didn't believe you could. In turn, build the strength and resilience required to go further in your health journey and everything you do.

The pleasure is all mine as I teach you how to work and seek out help when you recognize you need it. You will be better prepared to design workouts that you can engage with while having fun and being challenged.

At the same time, understand that your overall health reflects your thoughts, words, and beliefs. It's crucial to recognize that our inner dialogue shapes our reality. The thoughts we entertain, the words we speak, and the beliefs we have about ourselves can either empower us or limit us.

This book serves as a guide to help you cultivate a mindset that aligns with your true worth and potential as defined by God rather than the limiting narratives imposed by society or negative experiences.

With so much being covered in this book, no other topic is more important than the topic of God's love! He wants the best for you. He wants you to want the best for yourself, but it all starts with your thoughts.

Keeping the title of this book in mind, "Our Health & The Bible," the words we use about ourselves matter. So often, we self-inflict without realizing it. We forget that words have power. We must do a better job with how we use the tongue. Need an example? How's this:
*I'm so ugly
*I'm so fat
*I can't believe I ate that much today
*I'm such an embarrassment to my family
*Why can I stay consistent with my diet
*Forget it

If we think unhealthy thoughts, we'll say unhealthy things about ourselves. Our sayings become our everyday actions. Having a confident outlook on who you are and WHO you belong to (GOD) will give you a greater sense of purpose in life, which comes with a greater responsibility to care for our bodies from the inside out. This is where health begins.

Our health is not for ourselves. You see, Jesus came to serve, not to be served, and we are to be like Him.

So, our health is our responsibility to serve others in the best possible manner.

Not to overwork ourselves and be exhausted every day to begin shifting blame due to our lack of energy. We will learn to take accountability for our health and current state of mind. And I'll go even one step further: our attitude toward one another.

Have you ever done this before? Hit the snooze button ten times before getting up, only to realize you are running ten minutes late, making you twenty minutes late to work. When you finally arrive, you give a piece of your mind to two co-workers while ignoring the one who said, "Good Morning."

Our thoughts equal our behavior. Our actions equal our results. If we monitor what we think about, then our actions will always lead to greatness. And for what it's worth, we should *give* our bodies daily as a living sacrifice for God and as a benefit for others. We can't do much for others if we are in a hospital bed, sick, unable to do anything for ourselves. Failure then becomes what you believe about yourself. And that lie will become a cycle of misery that we don't need to live in.

Without the right mindset and healthy habits, you cannot test and approve God's good, pleasing, and perfect will because you will be so entrenched in your misery that you cannot discern His will.

BUT TAKE HEART

Physical activity, stress management, sleep routine, mind-body connection, prayer, and the will to make it all possible are in all of us. You will learn not to live in fear because it is a choice. The fear of rejection, fear of disappointment, fear of whatever it is that stops you from living your best life. The life God intended you to live is honest and full of life. Not convinced? Read John 10:10 with me out loud,

*"The thief comes only to steal and kill and destroy; I have come that they may have **life**, and have it to the full."*

Take your time reading this book and put everything you learn into action! Without action, you get no results.

I GOT YOU!

Chapter 1

Perception of Mindset

Many of us face this common struggle, and recognizing it is the first step toward change. We often carry burdens that don't belong to us, believing it's our duty to fix everything for everyone. This mindset can lead to overwhelming stress, fatigue, and feelings of isolation. But what if we changed our perspective? What if we recognized the difference between supporting someone and shouldering their weight?

It's essential to understand that you have limitations. You are not a superhero, and you can't solve every problem that arises in the lives of those around you. Acknowledging your limits is essential for maintaining your mental and emotional well-being. It's okay to say, "I can't take this on right now," or, "This is not my burden to bear."

Setting boundaries is essential for maintaining your mental health. It expresses, "I care about you, but I also care about myself." Establishing boundaries enables you to support others without losing yourself. You can be there for someone without adopting their struggles as your own.

While practicing self-care and supporting others, remember to recharge, participate in activities that bring you joy, and practice mindfulness. Self-care isn't selfish; it's essential. Taking care of yourself enables you to support your loved ones without feeling exhausted. It's easy to feel guilty for not being able to do more for others.

However, it's essential to let go of that guilt and understand that you are not responsible for someone else's happiness or outcomes. Each person has their own journey and challenges to overcome. Your role is to offer support, not to initiate their journey.

It's okay to express your feelings of overwhelm. Sharing your feelings with loved ones can foster deeper connections and open the door for mutual support. Vulnerability creates an environment where everyone feels safe sharing their struggles without judgment.

Don't forget to have regular check-ins with yourself about your intentions. Are you genuinely trying to help or seeking validation through your actions? Life is a delicate balance of giving and receiving support.

It's essential to find that equilibrium where you can be there for others while honoring your needs. Strive for harmony in your relationships, where parties feel valued and respected.

Remembering that it's okay to wake up feeling less than perfect is crucial. It's a part of being human. What matters is how we choose to respond to those feelings. By recognizing our limits, setting healthy boundaries, and supporting others without carrying their burdens, we create a more balanced and fulfilling life.

Let's embrace this journey together while encouraging one another to navigate the complexities of life and prioritize our well-being. We can learn to be there for each other without losing ourselves.

Let's start with work.

WORK

Most of us overextend our ability to do things. Then, we are stressed beyond our limits, causing us to feel overwhelmed and exhausted.

Why do we do it?

What will we gain from it?

Is it for a promotion?

Is it worth our health?

These questions, along with others, are what you should be asking yourself. You see, our place of work will always talk about work-life balance, and even if they don't, you should. You should not only talk about it but also *practice* work-life balance.

What does work-life balance look like for you? Let's be clear: I'm not saying to abandon your job; I'm not saying don't do your job. I'm not saying forget about your job. I'm telling you to balance your career and your home. Your work should never follow you home, and your personal issues should stay at home.

People often say separating the two is difficult, but that is far from the truth. It's all in the mind. That's right; it's your mindset and perception of things. Without a mental shift, things will never change, and a work-life balance will not be established.

SHIFT

What kind of shift, and how do I begin?

Two fundamental questions you may find asking yourself.

The answer is simple: it's an intentional mental shift.

This means becoming more aware of yourself and how you start the day. It's taking responsibility for what you feed your mind versus what you allow social media to feed it. But if you want to get a hold of an everyday work-life balance, you must read along.

Comfortability can be a double-edged sword.
While it provides a sense of security and familiarity, it often leads to complacency, where we stop striving for more. We settle into routines that may feel safe but do not challenge us to grow or explore our true potential. This comfort can create a false sense of achievement, making it easy to overlook the deeper desires and passions that lie within us.

When we become too comfortable, we risk stagnation. We may find ourselves just going through the motions, merely existing rather than truly living. It's essential to recognize that success demands stepping outside our comfort zones and embracing discomfort, as this often leads to growth, learning, and new opportunities.

Discomfort is a natural aspect of pushing boundaries and pursuing success. During these challenging moments, we uncover our true capabilities. Take time to reflect on what you genuinely want to achieve. Are your current actions aligned with your goals? Reassessing your objectives can reignite your motivation and help you break free from the cycle of comfort.

These goals should be ambitious but achievable, motivating you to take risks and invest the effort needed to reach them. As you pursue these goals, you will grow and evolve in ways you never imagined.

Embrace that failures and setbacks are valuable lessons, not dead ends. Take action. Comfort can often lead to inaction. To break this cycle, take small, deliberate steps toward your goals. Each step will strengthen your commitment to growth and success.

As you venture beyond your comfort zone and pursue your goals, celebrate even the most minor victories. Comfort will not lead you to the success you desire. Comfort is the foe of success.

"HOW?" I'm glad you asked.

Staying in a state of comfort will lead you to live a mediocre lifestyle. No one wants to realize or admit that our choices cause our lives to lack, and don't get me started with "age." Depending on an individual's "old age," we have to sit back and hear the complaints that come with age. We often don't take the time to work on our mindsets because we don't like.......*CHANGE.*

Change is not only necessary for us, but it will also benefit those around us. When you shift your mindset from wanting to do things your way to wanting to do things God's way, you no longer rely on your way of thinking to achieve things at work and home.

There's a quote that I read once that stated, "Do not conform to the patterns of this world but be transformed by the renewing of your mind" (Romans 12:2). This means NOT to stay comfortable with how you've been doing life. This quote encourages everyone to think twice before blending in and adapting to the ways of this world.

So, if we are not to conform to the ways of this world, then what are we to do? The second portion of that quote above states that renewing our minds should transform us. This means we must hit the RESET button in our lives to avoid feeling like we must take on every situation from every coworker or boss.

We would feel so much lighter in the mornings if we woke up leaving everything in God's hands rather than trying to devise a game plan for the day. Let me encourage you by saying this: not experiencing the shift will throw everything you are trying to accomplish off.

Most importantly, if we don't shift our mindset to a healthier one, we risk losing our way of thinking along with our joy, peace, hope, and kindness toward others. I understand what you're thinking: "Easier said than done."

Have you ever thought about what would happen if you never made the mental shift? If you never changed, what would life look like for you? Have you ever thought about that? Most people haven't.

Change can be difficult, but we can't allow it to stop our growth. Think about how much change happens around you daily; you don't even think about it; you adapt.

Let's start with the weather. Since 50% of us won't check or listen to the weather forecast before leaving the house, we assume by looking out the window that it will be a great day. The sky is clear of clouds, and it's just an ordinary sunny day. However, around noon, it starts to feel darker outside, as if someone is dimming the lights. Then, within seconds, you begin to hear thunder. The weather is changing; rain is on its way; you didn't prepare by grabbing an umbrella from the house, but guess what? You adapted.

It's time to leave work, and it's pouring out. You didn't say, "I'm going to stay clocked in at work until it stops raining." No. You found a clean trash bag (ladies), wrapped it around your head so as not to get your hair wet, and ran to your car. Men, you looked at the rain, said a few words under your breath, and dashed to the car. You adjusted.

You can also discern a person's true character by how they adapt and their mindset through their actions. Answer me this....DO YOU KNOW YOURSELF well enough to know how you would adjust to situations in life, or does life still get the best of you?

Who Are You?

I know I'm covering so much ground here because I aim to get you to expand your thinking. So, I ask again, who are you? In just one sentence or word, drop below who you are.....

_____

Before you answered the question on the previous page concerning who you are, did you think about it first? Or did you label yourself with the first word that came to mind? Here's a more profound question: before you thought about who you were, did you consult God? Did you check in with the Holy Spirit to see what He would have to say about you? It's ok if you didn't. We live such a fast-paced life that we often forget to pause to check in to see what God has to say concerning us. I'll give you a second chance to answer the same question............

Who Are You?

_____

_____

Some people can't answer the question. They go straight into their work title, church title, or who they are at home. But none of those titles genuinely define you.

The question, "Who Are You," is geared towards what you think about yourself and who you believe you are from the inside out.

Creating work-life boundaries wouldn't be difficult if you were secure and sure about who you were. Before we move on to Home and Social Life, we must know who we are in our hearts and minds so we are not found as double-minded men (male/female) as we progress. If you're unsure what a double-minded man consists of, let me share that with you now. According to the book of James 1:8, a double-minded man is unstable in ALL they do. So, you must know who you are unless you are like one who looks at himself in the mirror and forgets what he looks like when he walks away from it (James 1:23-24). Let us not be like that man.

Lastly, keep in mind whoever controls your mind controls you!

Chapter 2

Home and Social Life

How much *fun* is your home? Is it a place where you rush to get to? Or do you find yourself making unnecessary stops to bypass time? Home should be a sanctuary where laughter resonates, memories are created, and you can be yourself. For many, it has become a place that feels more like a pit stop than a joyful retreat. Assess your home's ambiance and consider whether or not it brings you joy or worry.

Take a moment to evaluate its energy. Is it filled with love, warmth, and laughter? Or does it feel tense and chaotic? The environment we cultivate in our homes profoundly affects our emotional and mental well-being.

Ask yourself, "When I walk through my front door, do I feel a sense of peace or overwhelmed and drained?" Consider how you feel in your home. Reflect on the emotions that arise when you think of home. Are they positive, or do they evoke feelings of stress and discomfort? It's crucial to bring awareness to your emotional state and understand what might contribute to these feelings.

The dynamics between the people in your home significantly affect how enjoyable and fun it is. Are your relationships filled with love, support, and laughter? Or is there tension, conflict, or a lack of communication? Ask yourself, "Do we genuinely enjoy each other's company, or do we often find ourselves avoiding meaningful interactions?"

Fun doesn't just happen; it's something we actively create. Think about the activities that bring joy to your household. Ask yourself, "What can I do to foster an atmosphere of fun and playfulness in our home?"

It's easy to let quality time slip away in our busy lives. Focus on activities that enhance your relationships and foster lasting memories. Consider this question: "When was the last time you had a meaningful conversation or felt joy?"

Change starts with sincere reflection and a commitment to turning your home into a space where everyone feels valued, loved, and eager to be. By embracing these challenges and taking actionable steps, you can cultivate a haven of joy and connection in your home.

This chapter seeks to shift you from a state of comfort to one of discomfort. You need to ask yourself some challenging questions to discover what your heart truly feels about your home.

Many of you attain different titles: father, mother, husband, wife, stepfather, stepmother, grandmother, grandfather, auntie, uncle, cousin, or child. But that's just the beginning of names. Many wear the title of chef, plumber, carpenter, mechanic, electrician, gardener, landscaper, and more after working a 9-5. How does that make you feel?

_____

_____

_____

_____

_____

_____

_____

_____

Many times, for men, there seems to be a greater pull on us since we are the head of the home. No matter how tired we may be after working all day, if the toilet needs fixing, we better jump on it. If the sink is clogged, we better unclog it. All while feeling or not feeling like it. And women alike. After working all day, coming home to tend to the children (if you have any), it doesn't stop there. Something always needs to be swept, mopped, or wiped down. Not to mention, dinner needs to be cooked, so how do you adjust?

The Bible calls for a husband and wife to become one. What does that look like in your home? Every home will look and feel different, let's be honest. There are only 24 hours a day, and when you put time into some titles, you take time away from others. Where is the balance? Is there a set schedule that says, "I will give my job eight hours a day, my children three hours a day, and my wife five hours a day?" Let's total that up; we're at 16 hours already for the day. That leaves us eight hours for self-care and rest. How is the balance in your home?

More time should be spent at home than outside. This would be fine unless there's a financial issue that requires overtime. However, aside from needing overtime, we cannot enjoy working on cars (men) more than we enjoy being home. Our absence is not suitable for the mental state of our wives. According to the Word of God, we ought to "live with our wives according to knowledge and with respect as the weaker partner" (1 Peter 3:7).

SAFE SPACE

Your home should be your safety. The place where you can lay your hair down (ladies) and men can walk around in their boxers (if there are no children in the home). Your home should be the place that prepares you to BECOME the person that God intended for you to become with prayer, fasting, and meditation.

Your home should be a place where you can speak freely without having to look over your shoulder to be judged. But a place where you are most heard and respected. Let's face it: some people are not disrespected until they come home. And that's a sad truth.

We must protect our homes. Coming home should feel like a breath of fresh air. We should be able to look at the person we are coming home to and think, "Man, I love this soul." Your home should never have to compete for your time, even with your social life.

SOCIAL LIFE

Having a well-balanced social life is KEY!
Do you feel like you don't get out often? Or are you someone who could slow down on your outings? Finding balance in our daily lives is essential for maintaining our mental and emotional well-being. Being confined within the same four walls—whether at work or home—can lead to stagnation and restlessness. Incorporating moments of freshness and change into our routines is crucial.
Nature has an incredible ability to rejuvenate our spirits. Make it a priority to step outside. Fresh air, sunlight, and the sights and sounds of nature can do wonders for your mood

and energy levels. Consider asking yourself: "When was the last time I took a moment to appreciate the outdoors?"

Social interactions can help break the cycle of routine. Reach out to friends, family, or colleagues for a chat, a meal, or an outing. Sharing experiences and laughter can lift your spirits and provide a fresh perspective. Ask yourself, "Who can I contact for quality outdoor time?"

I know that some people's co-workers become like family members because they live out of state and are away from their biological family members. We start calling our co-workers "Sis and Bro," and that's ok.

BUT.......

What happens when "Sis and/or Bro" is now being looked at for the promotion you were promised? If the relationship is not strong enough, you may begin to resent your "Sis/Bro" and can't say things like CONGRATULATIONS.
So, there must be boundaries set in place so we do not abuse relationships and friendships that were once God-sent. The people we connect with on a social level have to be people of value. Don't get me wrong, that's not a statement given to look down on anyone because each one is valuable in their own way.

But when it comes to self-growth, we must consider the people we keep in our backroom.
Let me explain the backroom.

It's a private space. It separates co-workers, friends, family members, and the best man or "bestie," as you women like to say. The back room is reserved for those who can handle your tough and personal conversations while trusting you'll never hear your conversation again from a third or fourth party that wasn't in the room. We all need friends that we can do more than talk to but vent to. Venting should be kept and designed only for a particular group of people.

It's important to understand that it's not all about one thing or another. It's simply about everything working in unison. Home, work, and life. It's the only way you'll be able to enjoy the things and people of this world while keeping a clear and healthy mental state. God even gave balance to plants and the trees of the field. They are provided with a certain amount of sunlight and water daily.

If God is faithful to bring balance and nourishment to the plants, trees of the field, and the birds of the air, how much more valuable are we to ensure our well-being (Matthew 6:26). Think about it. Your mental health matters to God.

So, you may be saying, "How do I reflect on and redirect my life so it mirrors more on focusing on the things that matter the most?

You ask great questions.

Reflection is next.

Chapter 3

Reflection with Self & God

You've developed resilience and the toughness to get through every trial and test. Each challenge you've faced has equipped you with tools to navigate the complexities of life. The struggles you've endured have tested your strength and refined your character, teaching you lessons that can only be learned through experience.

Sometimes, we have to peek back over our shoulders to understand that what we've gone through has made us who we are today. I can't imagine what it might look like over your shoulders, but I can assure you that what you've gone through or maybe even going through now has destroyed many people. But because you stand with such persistence, you can manage through.

Moreover, you have a support system, whether it be friends, family, or mentors, who have believed in you even when you doubted yourself. They have provided encouragement and wisdom, reminding you that you are not alone.

The ability to reflect and express gratitude, as you are doing now, is a powerful tool. It fosters a sense of contentment and peace, ensuring you remain grounded even in turbulent times. By recognizing your progress and the strength you've gained, you empower yourself to face whatever lies ahead with confidence and courage. As you continue your journey, remember that your challenges have not defined you but shaped you into a resilient individual capable of achieving great things.

Many people focus so much on the negativity surrounding them that they fail to realize they attract this negative energy through their thoughts. Since everything begins with an idea, we manifest what we constantly think about. Good or bad. People like yourself who focus more on the goodness of God tend to press through to the other side because we know, as the famous quote goes, "This too shall pass."

When you and I sit down to reflect and meditate for the day, we must be mindful not to focus on things that don't matter. We are guided through the Word of God to concentrate on matters from ABOVE and not earthly concerns. This can seem challenging for many. Listen, I understand. So much distracts us that we lose sight of what we cannot see (the things of the Spirit). However, to regain that focus, we must wake up each morning with a "Thank You, Lord" on our lips. It can be transformative if you and I contemplate God throughout the day.

I know what you are thinking, "I don't have time for all that. Who has time to sit and think about God all day while I have work to do? Or, we say things like, "I'm the driver in the car-pool lane; I must focus on the road." Or "I'm a babysitter. I run a daycare center with 30 kids every day; I don't have time for *stuff* like that."

BREATHE

All I want you to do is focus on yourself! You should know that God loves you and is eager to hear from you throughout the day. Here are some ways to stay connected with yourself while reflecting on God during the day.
Grab a pen and a notepad.

1. Daily Journaling: Take a few moments each day to write down your thoughts, feelings, and prayers. Reflect on how God has been present in your life and the blessings you've experienced. This can help you process your emotions and deepen your connection with Him.

2. Gratitude: Every morning or evening, write down three things you are grateful for. This simple practice shifts your focus to the positive aspects of your life and reminds you of God's goodness and provision.

3. Scripture Reflection: Select a verse or passage from the Bible that resonates with you. Take note of this and consider its meaning as the day unfolds. Reflect on how it relates to you and what God may be trying to convey to you through it.

4. Mindful Moments: Set reminders on your phone or notes around your space to pause and take a deep breath. Use these moments to pray, express gratitude, or acknowledge God's presence.

5. Pray as you Walk: Take a walk outdoors and use this time to pray and reflect on your surroundings. Notice the beauty of creation and how it reflects God's love and artistry. Allow the fresh air and nature to rejuvenate your spirit.

6. Playlist: Make a playlist of your favorite worship songs that uplift and inspire you. Enjoy the music during your commute or while doing chores, allowing it to elevate your spirit and draw you closer to God.

7. Kindness: Look for opportunities to serve others. Whether it's a kind word, a helping hand, or a simple smile, these acts reflect God's love and can create a deeper connection with Him as you embody His teachings.

8. Reflective Prayer: Before bed, take a moment to reflect on your day. Write down any challenges you faced, how you felt God's presence, and the lessons learned. This helps you process your experiences and prepares your heart for the next day.

9. Focus on Intentions: At the beginning of each day, set an intention of how you want to feel or what you want to focus on. Invite God into that intention, asking for guidance and strength to carry it out.

10. Silence and Solitude: Carve out time for silence to listen for God's voice. In the busyness of life, it's easy to miss His guidance. Spend a few moments quietly, allowing yourself to be still and present with Him.

By incorporating these practices into your daily routine, you can maintain a strong connection with yourself and God. Remember, He is always there, ready to listen and guide you through the highs and lows of life.

Did that list overwhelm you?
Do you need something a little simpler? No problem.
Let's simplify this for you even more.

Time with God using these simple and easy steps:
*Set an alarm 15 minutes earlier than usual to wake up.
-Go on YouTube and find a ten-minute meditation.

DO NOT stay lying in the bed. You could fall back asleep.
*After ten minutes of meditation, sit for five minutes to gather your thoughts and feelings.
-This will help to place you in a state of gratitude.
*Make your bed and brush your teeth.
*Greet your family and begin your day.
*Set a five-minute alarm during lunch break.
-This is set to remind you to take five minutes to sit and check in with yourself (How are you doing? Are your feelings intact? Is there anything you want to discuss with God)?
*After those five minutes, enjoy your lunch.
*After work, before heading home or picking up the children from daycare or school, sit in your car with a 5-minute timer.
*Let God know how grateful you are for keeping you safe throughout the first half of your day.
-After those five minutes, head to your following location with a smile, knowing God loves you.
*After cooking dinner and checking homework, and right before you go to bed, set another 10-minute alarm for self-reflection.
Take this time to review your day. Examine what went right and where things went wrong.
-Have a mental plan for how tomorrow will be different and better. Give God thanks for the day and sleep well.

I know this seems like a lot, but trust me, the more you do this, the more natural it will become as part of your day and life. And as you're doing this with intention, remember that God loves you. Your reflection time will turn to praise, and your praise can be done however you choose.

You can choose to praise and thank God in your thoughts, or you can express your praise out loud. You can praise Him while walking down the street, going up and down the stairs, or moving through the hallway to and from your office. Don't be surprised if tears start to roll down your face. That's a sign that you are aligning your spirit with the Holy Spirit, and He's confirming His presence with you. It's His way of reassuring you that "No weapon formed against you shall prosper" Isaiah 54:17.

The _HOW_ doesn't matter. What matters is that you praise and connect with Him daily.

When you make time for reflection a daily habit, you begin to notice an internal shift. Life will be more enjoyable; work will become pleasant; the people you didn't like before will become tolerable. This must be an everyday practice to live a healthier and fulfilled life.

Will this be easy? No.
Some days will seem better than others. But what helps is being mindful of what you think throughout your day and not allowing negative thoughts to hinder your progress or rule over your emotions. What you think creates an emotion in your heart that drives action in your life! Purposefully focusing on the goodness of God will place you in a position where no person, situation, or circumstance can bring you down unless you allow it. This occurs only through daily discipline in reflection with yourself and God.

No matter how long it takes to get this discipline fine-tuned, God will always be there to see you through. He saved us for moments like these. For that reason, He walks and talks with us through the Holy Spirit. He'll never leave or forsake you because he created you with purpose and success. Jeremiah 29:11 says, "For I know the plans I have for you," declares the Lord, "plans to prosper you and not to harm you, plans to give you hope and a future."

I know I've said it maybe once or twice, but God truly loves you. Keep reminding yourself of God's love, and you'll find keeping the discipline to seek and reflect on him easy. Understand that God has given you all you need to continue in life. It's all inside of you through the Spirit. God is great and greater than any issue you will ever encounter.

Every day is a chance to draw nearer to God. Remember, don't focus on the moments you've faltered, because we all fall short of God's glory. As long as it is called TODAY, rise up, pray, show gratitude, and keep moving forward.

I want you to do something before we move on. Reflect on all that God has done throughout the years for you. Think about those tight situations you never saw yourself getting out of. Then, all of a sudden, something happened that made you say, "WOW! How did that happen?" I want you to think about those moments. Greater WOWs are coming soon.

Chapter 4

Forgiveness

I've been told on multiple occasions by different people that it's hard to reflect on the goodness of God when they don't truly feel forgiven for the wrongs they've done in the past or the present. My usual response is, "Let it go," but I've learned that it's a phrase that's easier said than done. I've also encountered those who believe God is some genie in a bottle. Rub the bottle three times, and BOOM, your wishes come to life. These are people who often are found asking for things without showing any gratitude. A genie is merely a fictional character trapped inside a bottle. Whereas God is real, He is everywhere all at once.

Letting go of past mistakes and embracing forgiveness can be challenging in our spiritual journey. Many people carry the weight of guilt and shame, which can cloud their ability to recognize God's goodness. Acknowledging these feelings and realizing that they don't define us is essential.

Forgiveness, both from God and ourselves, is a process. Here are some steps that might help in navigating this journey:

1. Acknowledge Your Feelings: Recognize that feeling remorseful or ashamed is okay. These emotions are part of being human. Instead of suppressing them, allow yourself to sit with those feelings for a moment, understanding their origins.

2. Seek Understanding of God's Grace: Dive deeper into God's word for grace. God's love and forgiveness are not

contingent on our perfection. They are gifts freely given, regardless of our past. Reflect on scriptures that speak to God's mercy, such as Psalm 103:12, which reminds us that our sins are removed as far as the East is from the West.

3. Confession and Prayer: Confess your wrongs to God. This act of honesty can be liberating. Seek His forgiveness and find the strength to forgive yourself. Prayer can also provide a space to express your struggles and seek healing.

4. Embrace the Journey of Healing: Understand that forgiveness is a journey, not a destination. It may take time to feel entirely free from the burdens of guilt. Be patient with yourself and allow God to work in your heart.

5. Surround Yourself with Support: Share your struggles with trusted friends, family, or a spiritual mentor. They can offer encouragement and remind you of God's truth when you struggle to see it.

6. Focus on the Present: Instead of dwelling on past mistakes, redirect your attention to the present and future. Consider what steps you can take today to live in alignment with your values and to make amends if necessary. This proactive approach can help you feel empowered rather than trapped by your past.

7. Celebrate Progress: Acknowledge and celebrate the small victories. Each step you take toward healing and forgiveness is significant, and acknowledging your progress can help reinforce the idea that change is possible.

8. Practice Self-Compassion: Treat yourself with kindness and understanding as you would offer a friend. Remember that you are worthy of love and forgiveness from God and yourself.

9. Engage in Acts of Service: Sometimes, serving others can help us find perspective and heal our wounds. Engaging in acts of kindness can remind you of the goodness in the world and help you appreciate God's grace in action.

10. Remember God's Promises: Hold to the promises found in scripture about God's faithfulness and love. He desires you to be free from guilt and live in His grace.

Although letting go may seem simple, it requires intentional effort and grace. It is a process filled with ups and downs, but as you embrace God's love and forgiveness, the weight of past mistakes begins to lift, allowing you to reflect more freely on His goodness.

God knows you more deeply than you know yourself. He comprehends your thoughts, your actions, and what you will express. Yet, He loves you beyond words. I believe He does because He sent His only begotten Son to die for us. Stop chasing perfection, as it creates unnecessary pressure. When someone struggles to accept God's love and forgiveness, it's often because they haven't forgiven themselves.
Can you relate?

Learning to treat yourself with respect and love is the first step toward self-forgiveness. The issue is that while we serve and worship God, there is also the Prince of Darkness. Satan himself tries to enter people's minds and hearts and instill in them the belief that they are not worthy of forgiveness from this great God.

But what he speaks is his naïve language: LIES. We have allowed the enemy to tell us so many things. We believe lies, knowing they hold no weight or truth. You'll have to take yourself back to the beginning of time to snap out of this pool of lies that the enemy has placed you in. Not the time you were born naturally by your mother, but you'll have to go deeper, to the beginning of time when no one existed but God.

If you think this way, God reminds you that He called you even before your parents thought about coming together. God intentionally brought your parents together because He knew they would have the perfect DNA to create the version of you He envisioned when He thought about you. Accept God's forgiveness. He is intentional about you. He gave His only begotten Son to die for us all. And through His Son, we gain forgiveness. When you accept this gift, you can start looking at yourself as God sees you- His child!

As we endeavor to accept ourselves as children of God, we improve our well-being and transition to a healthier mental state. This enables us to serve our community better and allow the fruits of the Spirit to blossom within us.

What are the fruits of the Spirit?

Galatians 5:22-23

*Love
*Joy
*Peace
*Forbearance
*Kindness
*Goodness
*Faithfulness
*Gentleness
*Self-control

Living intentionally through the fruits of the Spirit will soften us and help us be more patient with ourselves and others—especially with those who are difficult to deal with and those who are less fortunate than we are.

While no individuals are more "special" than any other, you stand out from a large group of people struggling to find bread and water to eat and drink. Don't believe me? Take a walk or a drive to your nearest local bridge. Once you arrive, report back what you saw. The point is, while we are no better because that could have easily been one of us, we ought to be grateful that we are in a different state of mind that allows us to constantly make decisions beneficial to our health, well-being, and family. Only through God's grace and mercy do we get to go back and reflect while being mindful of where we used to be.

Accepting God's forgiveness requires complete surrender to ensure you never fall back into what you've been forgiven for. Surrender also entails letting go of your "To-Do" list to free yourself from unnecessary clutter.

It can be challenging when you see a list of things to do, and God says, "Turn that list over to me."
Can you do it?
Will you do it?
Most importantly, here is why you should do it.

Surrendering your list to God reestablishes His priority in your life. It's about making a list, checking it twice, and asking God to put everything in its proper perspective. This practice builds trust and strengthens the bond between you and God, helping to keep your life intact and your health in a stress-free environment.

Keep this one thing in mind, "If God be for you, who can be against you? Romans 8:3. When you accept yourself as God's child and His forgiveness over your life, serving and being good to people can be something you do. You must not get caught up with what the world, co-workers, or family members may have to say. People can be a trip sometimes, but they also have a valid point to play in our lives. Without them, our patience and growth could never be tested.

Here's the TRUE test!
Have you given or done something for someone, and they didn't say thank you? How did that make you feel? Did you feel as if you might have been taken advantage of? Did you feel like giving them a "piece" of your mind?

Now for a more profound question......

How about God?

God gives us a new day every time we wake up, and we don't say thank you to Him. Think about how that may make Him feel. Remember the many things He has forgiven us and the ways He's provided for us daily. Thinking about these things can start your morning prayer time with Him.

There's no set amount of time to sit in prayer, but the quality of the time matters. Make it imperative to spend time with God. As your relationship with God grows, so will the value of other relationships.

Remember the amount of forgiveness and patience God has given you, so in return, you can show grace and mercy to others, but that starts with knowing *WHO* you are.

Let us forgive one another as God has forgiven us.

Chapter 5

Who are You?

When people ask me who I am, I have a two-word answer: a creator. This often shocks people because they believe I am a name. I am more than just a name. I need you to understand this with a higher level of thinking.

To understand who I am, I had to do some investigation of my Father. While examining the history of my Father, I've learned that He was and is a creator, which is of no surprise to me as to where I get my creativity from.

My Father's mind holds no limit. This allows Him to imagine anything and speak it into existence; we call it manifestation today. My Father is such a creator that people still talk about Him and His work today.

By now, you may be wondering who my Father is.

My Father is the ONE who laid the foundation of the earth. He was here before time began. He lives out of time and has brought forth everything out of nothing except through his words. THE CREATOR! Let's go deeper. My Father, with His imagination, called everything to BE. Let me share with you a story about *The Beginning*.

1 In the beginning God created the heavens and the earth.

² Now the earth was formless and empty, darkness was over the surface of the deep, and the Spirit of God was hovering over the waters.

³ And God said, "Let there be light," and there was light.

⁴ God saw that the light was good, and he separated the
light from the darkness.

⁵ God called the light "day," and the darkness he called
"night." And there was evening, and there was
morning—the first day.

⁶ And God said, "Let there be a vault between the waters to
separate water from water."

⁷ So God made the vault and separated the water under the
vault from the water above it. And it was so.

⁸ God called the vault "sky." And there was evening, and
there was morning—the second day.

⁹ And God said, "Let the water under the sky be gathered to
one place, and let dry ground appear." And it was so.

¹⁰ God called the dry ground "land," and the gathered
waters he called "seas." And God saw that it was
good.

¹¹ Then God said, "Let the land produce vegetation: seed-
bearing plants and trees on the land that bear fruit with seed
in it, according to their various kinds." And it was so.

¹² The land produced vegetation: plants bearing seed
according to their kinds and trees bearing fruit with seed in
it according to their kinds. And God saw that it was good.

¹³ And there was evening, and there was morning—the
third day.

¹⁴ And God said, "Let there be lights in the vault of the sky to separate the day from the night, and let them serve as signs to mark sacred times, and days and years,

¹⁵ and let them be lights in the vault of the sky to give light on the earth." And it was so.

¹⁶ God made two great lights—the greater light to govern the day and the lesser light to govern the night. He also made the stars.

¹⁷ God set them in the vault of the sky to give light on the earth,

¹⁸ to govern the day and the night, and to separate light from darkness. And God saw that it was good.

¹⁹ And there was evening, and there was morning—the fourth day.

²⁰ And God said, "Let the water teem with living creatures, and let birds fly above the earth across the vault of the sky."

²¹ So God created the great creatures of the sea and every living thing with which the water teems and that moves about in it, according to their kinds, and every winged bird according to its kind. And God saw that it was good.

²² God blessed them and said, "Be fruitful and increase in number and fill the water in the seas, and let the birds increase on the earth."

²³ And there was evening, and there was morning—the fifth day.

²⁴ And God said, "Let the land produce living
creatures according to their kinds: the livestock, the
creatures that move along the ground, and the wild
animals, each according to its kind." And it was so.

²⁵ God made the wild animals according to their kinds, the
livestock according to their kinds, and all the creatures
that move along the ground according to their
kinds. And God saw that it was good.

**²⁶ Then God said, "Let us make mankind in our
image, in our likeness, so that they may rule over the
fish in the sea and the birds in the sky, over the
livestock and all the wild animals, and over all the
creatures that move along the ground."**

**²⁷ So God created mankind in his own image,
in the image of God he created them;
male and female he created them.**

**²⁸ God blessed them and said to them, "Be fruitful and
increase in number; fill the earth and subdue it. Rule
over the fish in the sea and the birds in the sky and over
every living creature that moves on the ground."**

²⁹ Then God said, "I give you every seed-bearing plant on
the face of the whole earth and every tree that has fruit with
seed in it. They will be yours for food.

³⁰ And to all the beasts of the earth and all the birds in the
sky and all the creatures that move along the ground—
everything that has the breath of life in it—I give every
green plant for food." And it was so.

³¹ God saw all that he had made, and it was very good. And there was evening, and there was morning— the sixth day (Genesis 1:1-31, NIV).

Now that you understand my Father better, do you see why you and I are more than just a name on a birth certificate? We are creators. We were created in the image and likeness of God. Everything He spoke into existence; if we believe and have faith, we too could bring forth things into being that were not.

Everything is possible for the one who believes (Mark 9:23), and that's how powerful we are.

Now that you better understand my Father, I can easily explain Who I Am.
I am a Child of God
I am a Creator
I am a Force
I am Strong
I am a Father
I am a Husband
I am a Friend
The next time someone asks you, "Who Are You?"
Don't just focus on your legal name and job title. Be willing to explore your answer more deeply. It won't make you seem like this "Holier Than Thou" person. It's simply where your thoughts should be. Maintain that focus as if it's something God wants you to consider.

Knowing you're a child of God will help you realize that God can do exceedingly above and beyond anything you can think or imagine (Ephesians 3:20). God's word does not come back void. You can stand and trust who He says you are. It's another easier-said-than-done moment.

33

It's funny for those with kids and those who remember being kids. We would listen to other people more than our parents. It's kind of what our children do today.
Why? I'll never know.

The truth is we, as adults, do it all the time.
We go to others without consulting God. We agree and jump on board with people we think speak from wisdom and experience but are not always God-sent. When we engage in conversations like that, it proves that we are still not too sure about who we are. I'm not saying anything's wrong with getting a second opinion on things, but I am saying that we ought to be more cautious with whom we consult first.

You are GREATER than you think. It's time to brainwash your mind with the absolute truth of who you are.
God wants to bless you beyond what your eyes see, and your imagination can imagine.

God loves you. Never forget it. Always remember Genesis 1:26: you were made to dominate and rule over the Earth. Find your WHY, and you'll begin to live an abundant life.

Who Are You?

_____

_____

_____

_____

_____

_____

Chapter 6

Who I Am

In 2005, I thanked God for such a wonderful gift while cradling my daughter in my arms. I then asked God to bless my wife and me with another child, hoping that it would be a happy, healthy baby boy. I know that if I don't ask, I won't receive.

"Ask, and it will be given to you; seek, and you will find; knock and the door will be opened to you."
Luke 11:9, so I asked.

I went about my business and kept doing what I needed to do, living life until 2007. My wife came to me and told me we were having our second child. I was overwhelmed with joy. I had the mindset of, "Lord, in my humble state, I've asked for a son, but even if it's not in your will for me to have a son, it's okay with me. I'm not going to worry or complain. Let thy will be done."

I left the matter in God's hands and walked away. Because of my faith, I knew I would get what I asked for. I don't believe God's word to be true, but I **know** God's word to be true. You will understand after you finish reading my story.

The hardest thing I had to do was trust that my wife was carrying our son. For some reason, during this time, I found myself surrounded by Christians who were asking the wrong questions. One in particular: What if it's not a boy? As much as that would irritate me, I had to stay in line with God and know that what I asked for, I would receive.

One day, my wife asked me, "Honey, what do you want to name our child?"

"His name will be Gabriel Michael Rodriguez," I said without any doubt or hesitation.

"Would you like to choose a girl's name just in case?"

My wife's question shocked me; I immediately told her, "There's no "just in case." His name is Gabriel Michael Rodriguez."

I was completely certain in my mind, heart, and soul that God would grant me what I requested. It didn't matter who believed in me for my son or who disagreed. What mattered was that my Father was giving me what I asked for, as my mind was focused on God and not on the opinions of those around me. I encouraged myself with daily affirmations. Repeatedly, I would say,
*My mind is strong
*I am a child of God
*Greater is He who is in me than he who is in the world
*No weapons formed against me shall not prosper

 The "What-If" people surrounded me. You know: What if it's another girl? What if you don't get what you want? What if your wife wants another little girl? And on and on it went. I needed to distance myself from those individuals to realize they weren't the real problem. It was the enemy (Satan) manipulating them to instill doubt in me and undermine my faith in God and His word.
Bible verse *3 John 1:2,* says that He wants us to prosper as our souls prosper. He wants us to be in good health because

good health means we can achieve God's plan for our lives. Nothing else can fill our minds when we direct our intentions toward Him.

One day, I was with my wife at a birthday party, and this woman said to me,

"Hey, I hear you're having another baby. That's awesome. Congratulations, *but* I heard you're praying for a boy. What if it's not a boy?"

As soon as she was done speaking, I stopped the enemy at that moment because he used this woman to try to make me doubt my Father. I told her in a Spirit-filled manner,

"If it's not a boy, I would love her the way I love my firstborn but because his name is Gabriel Michael Rodriguez, I know it's a boy."

After that, I walked away because when the enemy comes, he may use people you look up to, love, admire, and those in authority. And for what? To make you second-guess God. To make you second-guess who you are. When the enemy does that, you need to know how to answer. If you stand there and entertain the enemy, what you're saying is you don't believe that God is going to give you what you asked for. Walking away can be the strongest thing you do when the enemy tries to make you doubt.

A few months passed, and my wife and I were at an ultrasound appointment. The technician asked my wife,

"Do you want to know the sex of the baby?" My wife looked at me and asked,

"Do you want to know?"

I said, "I already know, but if you want to know, go ahead."

The technician turned to my wife and said, "It's a boy."

My wife was happy, and I stood there with an "I already knew" look.

My wife excitedly showed everyone the ultrasound pictures, saying, "It's a boy!" Some people even looked at me as if to say, "You're just lucky."

But it wasn't luck. I don't live my life based on luck; instead, I live my life on faith! Let my story encourage you. While others may doubt you remember, the level of your FAITH moves mountains. With God, anything is possible.

BUT WAIT.....
HERE COMES ROUND TWO

On our way to another doctor's appointment, my wife and I learned that she had placenta previa, which means the baby was positioned above the placenta. The placenta serves as the baby's food source, and little Gabriel Michael Rodriguez was blocking his source of nourishment.

My wife had to be on bed rest, lying on her side for months. To make matters worse, we were also informed that my wife could start bleeding at any time, and if we saw just a spot of blood, we'd have to rush to the hospital, only having a 20-minute window or else.

The doctor explained that *if* my wife started to hemorrhage during her C-section, I might have to choose between her and our son. The Holy Spirit seized my mouth and my voice; he wouldn't let me speak, so I nodded to let the doctor know I understood what he said. The doctor looked at me with a surprised look and proceeded to ask one more time,

"You understand what I said, right?"

I shook my head once more. I couldn't agree, so we continued with the rest of the appointment. We were leaving and heading to the car; my wife turned to me and said,

"How do you feel about what the doctor said? You had no words during the time of the appointment."

I told my wife, "I could not talk at the moment. But I asked God for a son, and before I asked God for a son, I prayed to have you first. I will be bringing you and our son home with me on that day."

My wife proceeded, "If it comes down to it, choose our son."

Neither of us had anything to say after that. I drove home and helped her get situated until I was sure she was okay. I entered an empty bedroom, closed the door, fell flat on my face, and cried. I don't know how long I cried. I couldn't do anything else. When I was finally able to speak, I said,

"Lord, I leave my wife and son in your hands. I cannot do anything about what's happening. I will mess up everything if I try. This is not for me to handle; only you can handle it. Thank you, Father. I love you and appreciate everything you do."

I praised Him for a while longer and then moved on about my day, but from that moment on, round two became harder. The enemy was coming after me in my mind. I was now the one having to do the grocery shopping. I had to pick up our daughter from my mother-in-law's house. I had to go and get my wife something to eat if she didn't want anything already in the house. Every time I left the house, the enemy tried to put it into my head: "What if I get back and she's gone, and I wasn't there to help her?"

I began to worry about my health. I could feel myself becoming stressed and overwhelmed at times. Round two was tough. I was trying to hold on to God while taking care of myself, my wife, our daughter, and our unborn son. I had to press even harder into God. I needed strength that could only come from above.

Every day, the thoughts of, "What if she dies? What if they both died?" continued to play in my thoughts and mind. I had to give it back to God and apologize constantly.

"Lord, I can't handle this. I'm sorry I took it off your hands, but I give it back to you here. Thank you for wanting to help and take care of this for me."

I had to say a short prayer every day throughout the day. Before going to bed, I would feel the sheets for blood in case my wife was hemorrhaging. I don't know how I slept some nights, but I spent much time checking on our daughter at night because she would need to get up to go to the restroom. This was the most challenging thing I've had to do. But I kept my mind on God because I could not do it alone. I didn't want to trust the life of my wife and unborn son in the hands of anyone else except God.

Negative and unsupportive thoughts were torturing me. It wouldn't seem to stop. Until one day, I had enough. The enemy did his usual and asked, "What if they died?" But this time was the last. I spoke to God and said, "Lord, if either of them or both of them die, I will NOT blame you. I will NOT stop worshipping and praising you because I know it's not what you want to happen. You said to be fruitful and multiply. This is me doing what you told me to do. Thank you. I love you, Father."

See, here was the problem: as long as the enemy knew I was afraid of losing my wife and or my son, he had his foot on my neck. He always had something on me that he could use to control me, even if it was for a moment. Once I told him I wasn't afraid and wouldn't blame God, I took back the power I allowed him to have. The enemy was very quiet after that encounter. But I knew he was lurking. There were still some weeks left.

It was time for another ultrasound appointment. Tension was high when the doctor turned to us and said, "The baby has to come out."

The doctor left the room and called the hospital to let them know we would be on our way. My wife was sitting in a recliner. Trying to wait for her to get up, I assisted her. The technician yelled at me to get our car ready. I looked at her and said, "I need my wife before I can leave." I know she was trying to help in such a heated moment. I had to let her know our car was right out front, ready for us to get in.

We were on our way to the hospital now. Upon arrival, two doctors were waiting for us by the emergency entrance. We've never met them before. But a wheelchair was present for my wife. They took her in. I needed to leave my wife for a second to find parking. When I returned, they sat me in a different room, separate from my wife.

You can only imagine how I was feeling at this moment. I wanted to be, no, I needed to be in the room with her. They told me in just a few moments, they would allow me in the room with her as soon as they finished preparing for her C-Section. I looked around for my wife's regular doctor but didn't see him. The two doctors who met us at the emergency entrance for the first time were the ones handling my wife.

Naturally, I was beginning to panic, but quickly, I looked up and said, "God, I believe you've placed the best people on the job for my wife. I won't worry."

A nurse assistant entered my room with scrubs for me to put on when, all of a sudden, I felt this overwhelming burden of "What-If." I knew then it was the enemy's last effort to take me down. I was beginning to fall into this *sad mode* with thoughts such as: What if you're a single dad of two?

The thought of possibly losing my wife or son, or both, was taunting me. I knew I had to shake it off and get into fight mode. I felt something wet coming down my face. I placed my fingers underneath my eye. TEARS? No, it can't be. I won't allow it. I looked to God in heaven and said out loud, "This is not for me to handle. I give this back to you, God. This is the last time I will allow these negative thoughts to enter my mind."

I thanked the Lord, dried my face, and walked into the operating room where my wife was. Everyone had such pleasant looks and smiles. All we were thinking about was the success of this baby being born. I sat next to my wife and had a flashback of when my daughter was born. I remember standing up, and just when I did that, they showed her to me. So, this time, I stood up for the same experience. While laughing and joking with my wife, trying to make light of the situation, I saw them pull my son out of my wife.

Speechless.

I was filled with awe at how much God loved me, and all I had to do was ask, and he gave me what I asked for: a baby boy. But wait, he's not breathing.

The way the doctors looked at my son, I knew something was off. My son was blue in the face. They believed he may not have been breathing while still in my wife's womb. How did they miss that? How did they not catch that?

They instantly picked him up like a wet noodle and started to perform (Cardiopulmonary resuscitation) CPR.
Although everyone was watching this take place with their own natural eyes, I saw this through my eyes of faith. If God could grant me a son, I knew he could grant me a living son. And let's not forget what I asked for initially.
Do you remember?

I asked God for a happy and healthy baby boy.
I never asked for a dead son.
I was not accepting death.

As they performed CPR on my son, my wife proceeded to ask the doctor, "Did you take the baby out? I don't hear the baby." You could tell the doctors were nervous, maybe even scared to answer. But they responded, "They're working on the baby right now. He's okay."

At that moment, it hit me. The fight is not over. I can't allow nonbelievers to answer for me, and I have to see them as nonbelievers because I don't know what they believe or who they believe in. This is my family, and I plan on bringing my wife and son home. My wife stated again,

"I don't hear the baby. Did you take him out? Is he okay?"

Without hesitation, I quickly answered her back,

"The baby is fine. He's just not crying."

I wasn't speaking from what my natural eyes were seeing. I was talking by FAITH. I couldn't imagine what my wife was feeling or thinking, not hearing the sound of her son's cry. After this, she asked five more times, "I don't hear the baby. Did you take him out? Is he okay?"

Every time before the doctors could answer, I said,

"He's fine, he's just not crying."

The doctor working on my son did what no parent ever wants to experience or witness; he stopped. He stopped working on our son. There was nothing more he could do. It looked like something out of a movie, and everything was now going in slow motion.

The nurse in the room with us also seemed concerned. When she looked at the doctor, I could feel in her eyes that she was yelling, "Don't stop." But the doctor began to remove his gloves. My wife asked one last time, "I don't hear the baby. He's not crying. Is he okay?"

The nurse looked at her watch to take note of the hour, which they thought was my son's death. Still holding on to my faith and God, I answered my wife one last time, "He's fine, just not crying."

When I said that to my wife this time, I felt something; it was like I knew the assignment for the doctors was over, and now it was time for God to step in and show out. I believed my God would do what these doctors couldn't do. While I was thinking this, my son's little arm went straight up in the air. Showing a clenched fist, and he started to cry.

Once again, God did not let me down.

As I conclude this chapter, I encourage you to ponder this: your mindset should be so resilient that no matter who or what surrounds you, they cannot persuade you to change. Nothing holds more power over you than God's word. Don't let anything or anyone matter more to you than His word. Sixteen years later, my son is still alive. No one can convince me that miracles don't happen. Keep the faith; nothing is impossible for our God to accomplish.

Chapter 7

What is dead in your life, let's bring it to life

Reflecting on our lives, we sense that many things have perished: our hopes, dreams, and goals. We've buried them deep within ourselves. At times, we fail to see how they can be revived. Reviving something that has been buried so deeply is such a challenge. It's hard enough to achieve a goal that has just been presented to us, let alone one that lies hidden within us. Like anything else, we must search for it and truly want it. We have to genuinely desire the outcome of this goal and not let anything stand in our way.

When we set a goal, it needs to be with the intentionality of achieving it to the desired end. Sometimes, those goals are vague and/or in vain. We must be intentional when it comes to our health and genuinely wanting the desired end result because when we start something, and then we stop, and we start something, and then we stop, we get to the point where we *stop.* We lose hope, don't desire it anymore, and now it's impossible.

We say things to ourselves like, "I can never lose weight. I can never get healthy." So, we see our goals as dead. But those goals and dreams, for some reason, continue to be in our minds. They continue to bother us, for lack of a better word.

We made 'Becoming Healthy' about individuals who only want to lose weight, tone their muscles, and look like models ready for a close-up picture. And that's not the truth.

Becoming healthier starts with your mindset.

You are emotionally healthy.

You are physically healthy.

You are spiritually healthy.

Review chapters 1-3 to grasp what it means to be healthy. Let me provide an example. My current goal is to become stronger. Stronger in the sense of being able to handle sufficient weight and make my body resilient enough to withstand the demands of life:

-The demands of being a husband

-The demands of being a dad

- The demands of work and all of these titles entail

My timeframe for achieving this is for the rest of my life. I'm not creating a goal that I need to accomplish or would desire to succeed quickly. This is my goal or one of them for as long as I live. So, my goal is simple, and it means so much to me, not because of myself but because of the people I serve.

One of the things we do is we make the mistake of thinking that our health is for us. I believe something different. My health is for God and the purpose of spreading His word, and it's also for God's people whom I was put on this earth to serve, whether at home, work, church, or anywhere.

I know you're thinking, if my health is not for me, and it's for God, then what about me? Well, here's the thing: our health is not for ourselves but benefits us. We reap being mentally, emotionally, physically, and spiritually healthy. How much better is it when you live with the fruits of the spirit of joy, peace, and love than living miserable, angry, irritated, and annoyed as if you don't like anybody? We say things like, "I don't like people," yet we work in a people-serving industry. Why do we do that to ourselves?

I would much rather live with love, joy, and peace because that makes for a healthier and much better lifestyle. It makes for a more evident mindset and tremendous and achievable goals. I'm not saying to live naïvely. Some of us will read this and think we should be naïve about what's happening around us.

If we're Christians, we're supposed to have a much better outlook in life because of who we are and who we belong to.

Goal setting

When it comes to creating a goal, we need to make it simple because we need to be able to look at this goal and say, "This is what I want." Your goal (if it's a fitness goal) can and should continue as a lifestyle.

Am I going to have vague goals? Absolutely not! I need to be specific. If I'm asking God for help, I need to be clear and tell Him, "I need your help. I want to be healthier and serve you well, Lord."

Take some time to sit back, relax, and review your goals. Reflect on what you want to achieve. Give yourself a longer timeframe—not because you might not achieve it, but to avoid making it so short that you become discouraged if you fall short. Instead, see this timeframe as an opportunity for growth and learning.

Set milestones that allow you to celebrate your progress, no matter how small. Recognize that setbacks can happen, but they do not constitute failures. As you reflect on your goals, visualize what achieving them looks and feels like. Create a vivid mental picture that inspires you to take action. Write down your goals and break them into manageable tasks that you can tackle daily or weekly. This will make the journey feel less overwhelming and keep you motivated.

Share your aspirations with others; accountability can often be a powerful motivator.

Remember, the journey to achieve your goals is as important as the destination. Enjoy the process, stay flexible, and keep pushing forward with determination and optimism. You can turn your dreams into reality, one step at a time.

Whatever your goals are, prepare to apply the work needed to accomplish them. This will take seeking and finding time within your busy schedule to achieve it. It doesn't have to get accomplished simultaneously every day, but you do have to work at it every day.

Remember, you'll need to make it achievable, not only the goal and the result but also the work being put into it. Don't be afraid to work on your goals after or before bed; as long as the job gets done, push forward to achieve the goal.

And please, DO NOT get caught up with those who say you can ONLY work on your goals between this hour and this hour. Don't be alarmed; those people may carry your same last name. Remember, they are not the ones that are going to *work* towards this goal.

I realize I went on a bit of a rant there, but one of my biggest pet peeves is when people say that you must 'work out' at a specific time to achieve the best results. The issue with that information is that not everyone can hit the gym or workout at that particular time every day. Instead, if you are focused on reaching a goal, let's say, a fitness goal, do this: on your calendar or To-Do list, put in the time you can commit daily to reaching this goal. Monitor yourself weekly to see your progress. You want to know what you've done or failed to do when you view your notes after two or three months.

We tend to look at the things we did not achieve as opposed to what we did. Don't let that be you. Remember to celebrate every milestone. Be proud of yourself.

Go harder without injuring yourself.

Don't Stop!

If the goal is something you truly desire, why should you stop moving forward? If you keep going, you'll be able to look back and identify what happened or ask yourself these questions to help push you along way:

*What happened?

 *What caused me not to reach my goal in the first three months?

*Was it the amount or lack of time I put into it?

 *Was it the timeframe? Bad timing?

No matter how many questions you have to ask yourself, bring out the pen and notepad and write your questions and concerns down. Find a way to fix them. Become a solution-driven person. Remember, this chapter is titled, "What is dead in your life, let's bring it to life."

Tackle the issue(s) that did not allow you to reach your goal(s) within the first three months. Were the mornings not a good fit for you? Did you realize you're not a morning person? Maybe you were trying to work out during your lunch break. Were there too many distractions that you didn't consider? How about the evenings right before bed? Did you find yourself too tired and just wanting to lie down and relax?

You have to look at these scenarios and do your best to make proper adjustments. Be okay with the changes that need to be made. Remember the end goal and your *why*.

Remember, these are only examples. Whatever your goal is, you can achieve it and make it happen. Make your goal a reality in your mind until other people can see it happening in your life.

Remember:

*Create goals that you can achieve

*Create goals that have meaning for your life

*Create goals that bring you the benefits you need while serving God and His people

This book is not only about your physical health and well-being. Your goals must also include mental, emotional, physical, and spiritual health.

God bless you!!

Chapter 8

Words to Remember

These words are meant to support not only your physical health but also your mental, emotional, and spiritual well-being. Let's get started. These are the words, their meaning, and my explanation.

1) **Routine**- A fixed program that does not change, and you do the same thing repeatedly.

Reading the meaning of this word is boring. This word is good and not so good at the same time. Let me explain. First, we need to create a routine. For example, choose what days throughout the week you will be working out and what time. When you start doing this, decide what body part or system (cardiovascular and muscular systems) you will work on. This will determine the exercises you will be performing. Remember to change your workout every 3 weeks so your body does not hit a plateau.

2) **Plateau**- Reaching a state of little or no change after a time of progress.

Think about what you do at the gym. That gym routine has stagnated if you can name everything you do daily. You hit a wall, a plateau. Plateaus are hard to get out of if you think they are. You are less likely to reach a plateau if you change your routine often. Something as simple as changing one or two exercises could make a difference.

Consider changing the amount of repetition for each movement every 3-weeks.

3) **Repetition**- Doing an exercise repeatedly.

Let's say you're doing pushups and start from the bottom position. When you push your body up to the top position, you've just completed one repetition or rep. You will now have 2, 3, and 4 reps as you continue. You now have one set if you stop at four or whatever number you decide to stop at.

4) **Set**- A group of repetitions.

Doing multiple sets is the idea behind performing exercises to help you achieve your physical, spiritual, mental, and emotional goals. The more you move your body, the easier it becomes.

5) **Goals**- An aim or desired result.

Have you set goals since reading Chapter Seven? If not, take a moment to review Chapter Seven and create a goal worth achieving. Ensure your physical goals connect with your spiritual, mental, and emotional goals. For example, your physical goal might be to move around more. While moving, you could talk to God, which may help you achieve greater mental and emotional stability.

6) **Exercises**- Activity requiring physical effort to sustain or improve health and fitness.

Notice its *activities* that require physical effort. You don't have to go to a gym; you only need to do an activity that requires physical effort.

Examples are climbing stairs, walking long distances, or doing anything other than your everyday routine. The type of activity you engage in is necessary, but what truly counts is that you are active.

Let me clarify: the activity's nature plays a role.

Remaining inactive for extended periods is unproductive. Instead, opt for activities that prompt you to stand, walk, or frequently adjust your position—whether that involves moving around or changing your elevation.

Incorporating movement is essential to any activity you choose.

We all have established routines that guide us throughout our day. We wake up, stretch, brush our teeth, shower, etc. A part of that morning routine should include prayer. We should take the first moments of our morning to talk to God and express our gratitude for being awake, along with anything else that comes to mind. This particular routine with God should remain consistent, as praying regularly will help us avoid reaching a plateau in our spiritual journey.

God breaks through plateaus like wet paper. Without God, we will not progress. Repetition in prayer will help us build our faith in God.

While there's nothing wrong with spending quiet time with God in your closet and kneeling for the rest of the day, all God asks is for you to communicate with Him throughout the day. No, you are not boring God with what you might consider meaningless words. He is our Father, and we can converse with Him just as we do with anyone we respect. The more time you spend praying, the more stability and clarity you will experience mentally and emotionally. Prayer is about multiple sets of repetitions throughout the day and week with God.

A simple thank you or telling Him how beautiful the sunlight or weather is isn't much to ask for. It's an honor to make the physical effort to move closer to God. Doing this will help us keep our minds on God, improving our mental health. Our mental health creates emotions that will increase the LOVE in our hearts for one another.

God doesn't expect perfection but wants us to work toward greatness. And I quote, "I can do all things through Christ who strengthens me." Philippians 4:13

Chapter 9

Let's Get Started

Welcome to the part of this book that most of us love to hate—working out! Whether you've been exercising for years or just started, you've probably realized one thing: getting up and moving is essential for a healthy life. But let me tell you, the most challenging part of working out isn't the exercises themselves; it's the mental challenge of just getting started.

Here's the good news: you don't need to be an expert or have fancy equipment to begin. All you need is the willingness to start where you are today with what you have. Don't worry about sets, reps, or the perfect combination of exercises. Those things can come later. For now, let's focus on one thing: **moving**.

Before we dive in, let me tell you about myself and why I'm the right person to guide you through this journey. I have over 20 years of experience as a fitness, group, and boot camp instructor. I've worked with individuals in resistance training with weights, resistance bands, suspension training, and body weight exercises. Whether in the gym, the park, at home, or anywhere we can meet—that became our workout space. My goal is to help people like you make fitness a part of your everyday life, no matter your current level. I've seen firsthand how starting small and staying consistent can lead to significant results, and I'm here to help you do just that.

So, let's get moving!

Exercise 1: Push-ups

Push-ups are one of the best exercises for building upper body strength. They target your chest, shoulders, and triceps and even engage your core. If you've never done push-ups before or you're not strong enough to do a full push-up, don't worry—there are modifications you can start with.

Beginner Option: Wall Push-ups

   1.   Stand facing a wall, about arm's length away.

   2.   Place your hands flat on the wall at shoulder height, shoulder-width apart.

   3.   Slowly bend your elbows and bring your chest closer to the wall, keeping your body straight and your core engaged.

   4.   Once your chest is close to the wall, push yourself back to the starting position by straightening your arms.

   5.   Repeat for the desired number of reps.

Intermediate Option: Incline Push-ups

   1.   Once comfortable with wall push-ups, try moving to an incline. You can use a sturdy chair, a bench, or a low table.

   2.   Place your hands on the edge of the surface, shoulder-width apart, and your feet on the floor behind you so your body forms a straight line.

   3.   Lower your chest toward the surface while keeping your body straight, then push back up.

4. Repeat for the desired number of reps.

Advanced Option: Floor Push-ups

1. Start in a plank position with your hands directly under your shoulders and your body in a straight line from head to toe.

2. Lower your chest to the floor, keeping your elbows close to your body.

3. Push back up to the starting position.

4. Repeat for the desired number of reps.

Tip: Progress from wall push-ups to incline and floor push-ups. It's all about building strength gradually!

Exercise 2: Overhead Press

The overhead press is excellent for building shoulder strength and improving mobility. You don't need weights to start; just practice the movement and build strength over time.

Beginner Option: No-Weight Overhead Press

1. Stand with your feet shoulder-width apart and your arms by your sides.

2. Slowly raise your arms above your head without forcing the movement. Only go as far as your shoulders allow.

3. Lower your arms back down to your sides.

4. Repeat for the desired number of reps.

Intermediate Option: Resistance Bands or Light Weights

1.   If you have any light dumbbells or resistance bands, use them to add resistance. Hold the dumbbells at shoulder height or stand on a resistance band, holding the ends in each hand.

2.   Slowly press the weights or bands upward until your arms are extended.

3.   Lower them back down to shoulder height.

4.   Repeat for the desired number of reps.

Tip: If you experience shoulder pain or difficulty with this movement, see a physical therapist to assess your mobility and help you progress safely.

Exercise 3: Squats

Squats are fundamental for building lower body strength and improving balance. They work your quads, hamstrings, and glutes and even engage your core. If you have knee pain or difficulty with squats, there are ways to modify them.

Beginner Option: Assisted Squats

1.   Stand before a chair or sturdy object (like a countertop or broom handle) to hold on to for balance.

2.   Place your feet shoulder-width apart with your toes slightly pointing outward.

3.   Slowly bend your knees and lower your hips as if you're going to sit down in a chair. Stop if you feel pain or discomfort.

4.   Push through your heels and return to a standing position.

5.   Repeat for the desired number of reps.

Intermediate Option: Bodyweight Squats

1.   Stand with your feet shoulder-width apart, toes slightly turned out.

2.   Lower yourself by bending at the knees and hips like sitting in an imaginary chair.

3.   Keep your chest up, and make sure your knees don't go past your toes.

4.   Push through your heels to return to standing.

5.   Repeat for the desired number of reps.

Tip: If needed, start with shallow squats, then work deeper as you build strength. If you need assistance with balance, hold on to a chair for support.

Exercise 4: Crunches

Crunches are a simple yet effective way to strengthen your core, especially your abdominal muscles.

Beginner Option: Basic Crunches

1.   Lie on your back with your knees bent and feet flat on the floor.

2.   Place your hands lightly behind your head, making sure not to pull on your neck.

3.   Engage your core and slowly lift your shoulder blades off the floor, lifting your chin slightly and pointing toward the ceiling.

4.   Lower back down to the starting position.

5.   Repeat for the desired number of reps.

Tip: Maintain steady movements and avoid pulling on your neck. Focus on using your abdominal muscles to lift your upper body.

Progressing and Setting Goals

Now that you have a foundation of basic exercises setting realistic goals and tracking your progress is essential. Start with small, manageable sets and reps, such as:

•   Beginner: 3 sets of 5 reps for each exercise, three days a week.

•   Intermediate: 3 sets of 8–10 reps for each exercise, 3–4 days a week.

•   Advanced: 4–5 sets of 12–15 reps, with added resistance, 4–5 days a week.

You can gradually increase your reps, sets, or resistance as you become stronger. Pay attention to your body's signals— if you experience pain (not soreness), stop and evaluate whether you're performing the movement correctly or if you need to make adjustments.

Pain and Injury Guidance: Understanding Your Body

One of the biggest challenges in fitness is knowing when to push through discomfort and when to stop. Understanding the difference between the "good" pain of working muscles and the "bad" pain that could signal injury is important. This will help you make smarter decisions in your workouts and keep you on track to reaching your goals.

Good Pain: Muscle Soreness (DOMS)

After a workout, especially if you're new to exercising or trying a new routine, you might experience soreness. This is called Delayed Onset Muscle Soreness (DOMS), and it's completely normal. DOMS occurs when your muscles adapt to new stress levels, leading to tiny micro-tears in the muscle fibers. Your body then repairs these tears, which strengthens your muscles.

What DOMS Feels Like:

• A dull, aching soreness in the muscles you worked out

• Stiffness that sets in 12-24 hours after the workout and can last up to 72 hours

• Discomfort when using those muscles, but no sharp or stabbing pain

How to Manage DOMS:

• Gentle movement: Light exercise, walking, and stretching can help reduce stiffness

• Hydration and nutrition: Drink plenty of water. Eat protein-rich foods to help your muscles recover

• Rest: Give your muscles time to repair by allowing at least 48 hours before working the same muscle group again.

Soreness indicates that you're challenging your muscles. However, if the soreness becomes unbearable or doesn't improve over time, it may indicate that you have overexerted yourself, and you should take a step back.

Bad Pain: Injury Warning Signs

While muscle soreness is normal, pain that signals an injury should never be ignored.

What Injury Pain Feels Like:

- Sharp, stabbing pain during or immediately after exercise

- Swelling, redness, or warmth around a joint or muscle

- Inability to move a joint through its full range of motion

- Weakness or instability in a limb (e.g., feeling like your knee might "give out")

- Numbness, tingling, or radiating pain

If you experience any of these symptoms, stop your workout immediately. Continuing to push through could make the injury worse. Rest and assess the situation before continuing.

When to Seek Professional Help

If the pain doesn't go away with rest, ice, or over-the-counter pain relief, then it may be best to seek help from a healthcare professional. A physical therapist can help you understand whether your pain is due to a temporary strain or something more serious, like a tear or injury.

Examples of when to see a physical therapist or doctor:

• Persistent pain that lasts longer than a few days, even with rest

• Pain that worsens with movement

• Loss of mobility or strength in a joint or muscle group

• Unexplained swelling or bruising

Don't wait too long before getting help—early treatment can prevent a minor issue from becoming major.

Pushing Through Discomfort: The Right Way

Now that you know the difference between soreness and injury, let's discuss how to push through discomfort safely.

Here's how to push through the right kind of discomfort:

1. Modify the exercise: If a movement is challenging, adjust it. For instance, if full push-ups cause discomfort, try doing wall or incline push-ups instead.

2. Listen to your body: You should feel challenged but not in pain. If you feel a sharp or stabbing pain, stop immediately. You're likely in the safe zone if you feel a dull burn in your muscles.

3. Rest and recover: Rest days are just as important as workout days. Your muscles require time to recover and gain strength. Aim for at least one or two rest days each week, especially if you're just starting out.

4. Gradually increase intensity: Don't jump into heavy weights or advanced exercises too quickly. Allow your body time to adapt to the demands you're

putting on it. Gradual progression will help you prevent injury.

Building a Safe and Sustainable Fitness Routine

You will establish a challenging yet sustainable routine by understanding the distinction between beneficial pain and pain from an injury. Don't be afraid to take it slow and listen to your body—it's better to make steady, consistent progress than to rush and get sidelined by injury. Remember, the goal is not to push yourself to the point of pain but to challenge your muscles to grow stronger. With time and patience, your body will become more resilient and capable of handling the workouts you set out to do.

Setting Up Your Workout Routine

Now that you understand the exercises and how to manage pain and injury, let's talk about setting up a workout routine that works for you. The most important thing to remember is to *start where you are, not where you think you should be*.

Your fitness journey is personal, and the only way to make lasting progress is to create a routine that fits your current ability and goals.

We will start with a simple, foundational plan that progresses over time. This plan will give you structure while allowing you to modify it based on how your body responds.

Visit my YouTube channel, *@BarBellBelievers*, for more encouraging and detailed explanations of exercises. There, you'll find videos that can help guide you through each step of your fitness journey.

Understanding Weights: Heavy vs. Light

Before diving into the workout plans, it's important to grasp the distinction between heavy and lighter weights and how each can assist you in achieving different goals.

• Heavy Weights for Strength and Muscle Mass.

• If you aim to build strength and muscle mass, you should focus on lifting heavier weights with fewer repetitions (typically 6–8 reps per set). Heavyweights challenge your muscles and cause them to grow larger and stronger as they adapt to the increased resistance.

This approach is ideal for gaining size and improving raw strength.

• Example: If you can squat 50 lbs for 8 reps and it feels challenging by the last rep, you're using a weight appropriate for building strength and muscle mass.

• Lighter Weights for Muscle Tone and Fat Burning:

• If you aim to build muscle tone, increase endurance, and burn fat, lighter weights with higher repetitions (typically 12–15 reps per set) are more effective. Lighter weights allow you to complete more reps and keep your muscles under tension longer. This will help to boost your metabolism, improve muscle definition, and burn more calories.

• This method is effective for attaining a leaner body, focusing on muscular endurance and fat loss rather than developing substantial muscle mass.

- Example: If you use a resistance band or 5-lb dumbbells and complete 15 reps without feeling exhausted, you're in the right range for toning and fat burning.

Which One is Right for You?

- If you're starting out or looking to enhance your overall fitness and lose fat, begin with lighter weights or bodyweight exercises. As you progress, you can increase the repetitions and gradually add resistance.

- If your goal is to build muscle mass and enhance strength, increase the weights you lift as you grow stronger.

Start where you are, and remember that, depending on your goals, lighter and heavier weights can be part of your fitness routine.

Beginner Workout Plan (Weeks 1-4)

This plan is designed for beginners or individuals with physical limitations or discomfort. It emphasizes building a habit, gradually increasing strength, and preventing injuries.

Frequency: 3 days a week (Monday, Wednesday, Friday)

Workout:

- **Day 1**:

- Squats: 3 sets of 8 reps

- Push-ups (wall or incline): 3 sets of 5 reps

- Crunches: 3 sets of 8 reps

- **Day 2**:

  - Overhead Press (no weight or light weights): 3 sets of 5 reps

    - Squats (assisted if needed): 3 sets of 8 reps

    - Push-ups (wall or incline): 3 sets of 5 reps

  - **Day 3**:

  - Push-ups (wall or incline): 3 sets of 5 reps

    - Crunches: 3 sets of 8 reps

    - Squats: 3 sets of 8 reps

The goal is to focus on form and consistency. Don't worry if the reps seem low—this is about building a solid foundation. If you feel any discomfort, modify the movements or reduce the number of reps.

Intermediate Workout Plan (Weeks 5-8)

After four weeks, you'll likely notice that the exercises are becoming more manageable. This is a good sign that your muscles are getting stronger. Now, it's time to increase the challenge slightly by adding more reps and introducing light resistance (such as dumbbells or resistance bands).

Frequency: 4 days a week (Monday, Tuesday, Thursday, Friday)

Workout:

- **Day 1**:

  - Squats: 4 sets of 10 reps

    - Push-ups (incline or floor): 4 sets of 8 reps

- Crunches: 4 sets of 10 reps

- **Day 2**:

- Overhead Press (light weights or resistance band): 4 sets of 8 reps

- Squats: 4 sets of 10 reps

- Push-ups (incline or floor): 4 sets of 8 reps

- **Day 3**:

- Push-ups (incline or floor): 4 sets of 8 reps

- Crunches: 4 sets of 10 reps

- Squats: 4 sets of 10 reps

- **Day 4**:

- Overhead Press (light weights or resistance band): 4 sets of 8 reps

- Crunches: 4 sets of 10 reps

- Squats: 4 sets of 10 reps

Goal: Gradually increase your reps and sets. If you're feeling comfortable, add resistance. If you're using weights, start light and focus on maintaining proper form throughout each movement (2-5lbs).

Advanced Workout Plan (Weeks 9-12)

At this stage, you're building strength and endurance. You'll add more reps, sets, and resistance and might find that you can challenge yourself in new ways. It's important to keep listening to your body, but feel free to push a little harder now that you've built a solid base.

Frequency: 4-5 days a week (Monday, Tuesday, Thursday, Friday, optional Saturday)

Workout:

- **Day 1**:

- Squats: 5 sets of 12 reps (use weights if you're ready)

- Push-ups (floor): 5 sets of 10 reps

- Crunches: 5 sets of 12 reps

- **Day 2**:

- Overhead Press (heavier weights or bands): 5 sets of 10 reps

- Squats: 5 sets of 12 reps (use weights)

- Push-ups (floor): 5 sets of 10 reps

- **Day 3**:

- Push-ups (floor): 5 sets of 10 reps

- Crunches: 5 sets of 12 reps

- Squats: 5 sets of 12 reps (use weights)

- **Day 4**:

- Overhead Press (heavier weights or bands): 5 sets of 10 reps

- Crunches: 5 sets of 12 reps

- Squats: 5 sets of 12 reps (use weights)

- **Optional Day 5**:

- Choose two exercises (Push-ups and Squats) and do four sets of 12-15 reps each.

Goal: At this level, you're building muscle and endurance. The key is consistency and using the proper form to increase resistance. Take breaks when needed and listen to your body to avoid overtraining.

Tracking Progress and Adjusting the Plan

It's essential to track your progress and make adjustments as necessary throughout this 12-week program.

Here's how to make sure you're moving forward:

1. Keep a Workout Log: Write down how many sets, reps, and weights (if applicable) you use. This will help you see improvements over time and keep you motivated.

2. Adjust: If a particular exercise becomes too easy, increase the resistance or add more reps. If an exercise feels too difficult or causes discomfort, modify it or reduce the intensity.

3. Set Mini Goals: Set goals for each week or month, such as increasing your push-up reps or squatting deeper with good form. These small victories will keep you focused and motivated.

4. Rest and Recovery: Don't forget that rest is crucial for progress. If you're feeling sore, tired, or need a break, take a rest day. Your body will thank you, and you'll come back stronger.

Final Thoughts on Building a Sustainable Routine

Remember, fitness is a lifelong journey. There's no rush to complete multiple reps or lift a specific weight. What matters most is that you're making progress. Celebrate every victory, stay consistent, and trust the process.

As time passes, your strength, endurance, and confidence will grow, and you'll discover that what once felt impossible has become a part of your daily routine.

For further encouragement on your health journey, check out my YouTube channel, @BarBellBelievers.

I provide tips, motivation, and guidance to help you stay on track.

"Commit to the Lord whatever you do, and He will establish your plans." Proverbs 16:3

Chapter 10

The Power of Rest and Recovery

We often underestimate the role recovery plays in our fitness journeys. The truth is that muscles don't grow during the workout; they grow during the subsequent rest. When we engage in strenuous exercise, we create micro-tears in our muscle fibers. During recovery, these tears heal, increasing strength and muscle mass. Therefore, understanding how to incorporate rest days into your routine properly can make a difference in achieving your fitness goals. One key aspect of recovery is active recovery, which involves low-intensity activities. These can include walking, swimming, or even light yoga.

Active recovery promotes blood flow to the muscles, aiding healing, reducing soreness, and preventing sluggishness. Incorporating stretching and mobility exercises into your routine is essential for maintaining flexibility and preventing injuries. Stretching helps elongate tight muscles, improve range of motion, and enhance overall performance.

Mobility exercises that focus on joint movement and stability can also help identify and correct any imbalances in the body. Prioritizing these practices, you create a strong foundation for more effective workouts while minimizing the risk of injury. Sleep, often overlooked, is another vital component of recovery. Quality sleep is essential for hormone regulation, muscle repair, and cognitive function. During deep sleep, growth hormone is released, which plays a significant role in muscle growth and fat loss.

Aim for 7-9 hours of quality sleep each night to ensure your body has the time to recover and perform at its best.

While the grind and hustle of intense workouts are crucial, they must be balanced with adequate rest and recovery. By acknowledging the importance of recovery, utilizing active recovery techniques, stretching, and resting, you can prepare your body for the challenges ahead. Remember, fitness is not only about the effort you invest during workouts; it's just as much about how well you care for your body afterward. Embrace recovery as a vital part of your fitness journey, and you'll notice improvements in your performance and overall well-being.

Why Rest and Recovery Are Crucial

The Benefits of Recovery:

1. Muscle Repair: During rest, your body repairs damaged muscle fibers, making them stronger and more capable of handling future workouts.

2. Preventing Injury: Skipping rest days increases the risk of injury. Your muscles, joints, and ligaments need time to recover to avoid strains, sprains, and overuse injuries.

3. Mental Recovery: Exercise isn't just physically taxing; it's also mentally demanding. Rest days allow your mind to recover, helping you stay motivated and focused.

4. Improved Performance: Adequate rest leads to better gym performance. After a good rest day, your energy levels will be higher, and you'll be able to lift heavier or run faster.

The Role of Stretching and Mobility

Rest doesn't simply mean lounging on the couch all day. Participating in active recovery, such as stretching and mobility exercises, can improve flexibility, prevent injuries, and speed up recovery.

Why Stretching Matters:

1. Improves Flexibility: Stretching lengthens your muscles and enhances your range of motion. This is particularly important when lifting weights or engaging in strength training. Tight muscles can restrict your movement and raise your risk of injury.

2. Reduced Muscle Stiffness: Stretching after a workout relieves muscle tension, lessening the stiffness and soreness you may experience the following day.

3. Posture: Poor flexibility can lead to muscle imbalances, affecting posture. Stretching regularly helps keep the body aligned.

Types of Stretching:

Dynamic stretching involves moving your muscles through their full range of motion, making it ideal for warming up before a workout. Consider movements such as leg swings, arm circles, or walking lunges. Static stretching involves holding a stretch for 20–30 seconds to lengthen the muscle. It's best done after a workout to help with recovery. Examples include hamstring, quad, and shoulder stretches.

The Importance of Mobility Work:

Mobility exercises aim to improve the range of motion in your joints. They enable your body to move more freely and efficiently, reducing the risk of injury while improving your performance in squats, deadlifts, and overhead lift presses.

Simple Mobility Exercises:

1. Hip Circles: Stand with your feet shoulder-width apart and move your hips in a circular motion. This loosens up your hips, which is essential for exercises like squats.

2. Cat-Cow Stretch: Get on your hands and knees, arch your back toward the ceiling (like a cat), then lower it down, letting your belly drop (like a cow). This helps improve spinal mobility.

3. Ankle Circles: To improve ankle mobility, move your foot in circles. This is essential for exercises like lunges and squats.

Incorporating stretching and mobility work into your rest days ensures your body stays limber, flexible, and ready for the next workout.

The Importance of Sleep in Recovery

While stretching and rest days are essential, sleep forms the foundation of recovery. Your body does most of its repair while you're sleeping. If you're not getting enough quality rest, your progress will be limited—regardless of how hard you work in the gym.

How Sleep Affects Recovery:

1. Muscle Repair: During deep sleep, your body releases growth hormones that help repair and build muscle tissue. Without adequate sleep, this repair process is slowed down, affecting your strength and endurance.

2. Energy Restoration: Sleep restores energy levels by replenishing the body's glycogen stores, which is the fuel your muscles need during exercise.

3. Cognitive Function: Sleep also impacts your mental sharpness and focus. If you do not get enough sleep, your workouts will decline because your mind and body won't sync.

4. Sleep lowers inflammation in the body.

How Much Sleep Do You Need?

Most adults need 7-9 hours of sleep per night for optimal recovery. If you're training intensely, you may need even more. To prioritize good sleep hygiene, follow a regular schedule, create a relaxing bedtime routine, and minimize screen time before bed.

Signs You Need a Break

Overtraining can sneak up on you if you aren't careful. While dedication to your fitness goals is fantastic, there are unmistakable signs that your body may need more rest. Ignoring these signs can result in injury, burnout, or a plateau in your progress.

Here are some signs you may need a break:

1. Persistent Fatigue: If you're constantly tired, even after a full night of sleep, it could be a sign that you're overtraining and not giving your body enough time to recover.

2. Decreased Performance: If your strength, endurance, or overall performance declines, it's a clear sign that your body needs more rest.

3. Irritability or Mood Swings: Overtraining affects your body and mind. Feeling unusually irritable or stressed could be a sign that your nervous system is overworked.

4. Aches and Pains: Persistent aches, especially in your joints or muscles, could mean you're pushing too hard. This pain is different from normal soreness and shouldn't be ignored.

5. Lack of Motivation: Dreading your workouts or feeling unmotivated to exercise could be a sign of burnout.

6. Sleep Issues: Overtraining can result in difficulty sleeping, which creates a vicious cycle of inadequate recovery.

If you notice any of these signs, it's time to take a break. Rest focus on recovery, and return feeling refreshed. Sometimes, a few days off is just what your body needs to recharge and rejuvenate.

Conclusion

Rest and recovery are not optional; they are essential for progress. Whether you give your muscles time to repair, stretch to enhance mobility, or get quality sleep to replenish your body's energy, recovery is the foundation that supports everything you do in the gym.

Remember, your body is a machine—it needs regular maintenance to perform at its best.

Listen to your body if you feel fatigued, unmotivated, or in pain. Take a break when needed, prioritize rest, and make recovery a regular fitness routine. By doing so, you'll ensure that every time you step into the gym, you're ready to give your best.

Book Recap

Chapter 1: Perception of Mindset

Your mindset shapes every aspect of your life, including your health and wellness. This chapter reminds you that the weight you feel daily is often due to the burdens you decide to carry. It's about letting go of the need to control everything and focusing instead on balancing work, home, and self-care. Remember, a renewed mind is the first step toward living a healthier, more fulfilled life.

Chapter 2: Home and Social Life

Your home should be your sanctuary, a place where you can recharge. This chapter encourages you to consider how you balance your time with the people closest to you. It's not just about managing responsibilities; it's about prioritizing your home life above all else to create a foundation of peace and support. Your relationships at home are vital to your mental and emotional health.

Chapter 3: Reflection with Self & God

Daily reflection is vital for spiritual, mental, and physical well-being. In this chapter, you are encouraged to pause and appreciate your current state by reflecting on God's grace. Focusing on God's goodness rather than life's challenges can transform how you approach every situation. By staying connected with God throughout your day, you will discover strength, clarity, and peace in all aspects of your life.

Chapter 4: Forgiveness

Forgiveness is a cornerstone of spiritual and mental health, yet it's often one of the hardest things to accept.

This chapter is about letting go of guilt and truly accepting God's forgiveness, allowing you to heal and move forward. Forgiving yourself frees you to offer that same grace to others. Start by accepting God's love for you, and you'll see how much it transforms your life and relationships.

Chapter 5: Who Are You?

Who are you? It's a more profound question than just your name or job title. This chapter challenges you to think about your identity as a creator, as someone made in God's image. When you understand your identity in God's eyes, you can confidently step into your purpose with clarity, embracing the power He has given you to create, lead, and inspire.

Chapter 6: Who I Am

I share a personal story about faith, persistence, and the power of belief. It reminds you that your mindset and faith greatly influence your life's outcomes.

No matter the circumstances or the voices of doubt around you, miracles can happen when you believe in God's promises and stay focused. It's about knowing who you are and standing firm in that truth.

Chapter 7: What is Dead in Your Life, Let's Bring It to Life

Many of us feel our dreams or goals are long dead, but this chapter reminds us that nothing is truly lost. It's time to revive those desires for health, relationships, or personal growth by intentionally setting realistic, meaningful goals; you can bring life to those forgotten parts of yourself. It's never too late to start fresh; your health is the beginning of a renewed you.

Chapter 8: Words to Remember

Before diving into a workout routine, this chapter teaches the power of routine, breaking plateaus, and staying motivated. It reminds you that consistency in your physical, spiritual, and emotional efforts will lead to long-term growth. Every repetition, set, and prayer builds your strength—not just physically but mentally and spiritually. Your routine with God is as essential as your time in the gym.

Chapter 9: Let's Get Started

This chapter focuses on taking the first step toward physical activity, regardless of your fitness level. It emphasizes that perfection isn't necessary, and you don't need to know everything about the rules.

Begin where you are and prioritize building consistency. The chapter offers simple exercises and encourages you to do what you can without rushing, understanding that progress unfolds over time. It serves as a reminder that your fitness journey is a process, and starting small is still a start!

Chapter 10: The Power of Rest and Recovery

If you did not take anything out of this chapter, let this be one of the key lessons learned: Rest and recovery are **not** optional; they're essential for progress. May you find rest as you pursue your goals and dreams.

THANK YOU!

www.ingramcontent.com/pod-product-compliance
Lightning Source LLC
Chambersburg PA
CBHW070753003326
4I9I4CB00053B/736